A New Mother's Guide

POST PREGNANCY DIET
The Secret Recipes For New Mom

AMY TAN

Text Copyright © Author

All rights reserved. No part of this guide may be reproduced in any form without permission in writing from the publisher except in the case of brief quotations embodied in critical articles or reviews.

Legal & Disclaimer

The information contained in this book is not designed to replace or take the place of any form of medicine or professional medical advice. The information in this book has been provided for educational and entertainment purposes only.

The information contained in this book has been compiled from sources deemed reliable, and it is accurate to the best of the Author's knowledge; however, the Author cannot guarantee its accuracy and validity and cannot be held liable for any errors or omissions. Changes are periodically made to this book. You must consult your doctor or get professional medical advice before using any of the suggested remedies, techniques, or information in this book.

Upon using the information contained in this book, you agree to hold harmless the Author from and against any damages, costs, and expenses, including any legal fees potentially resulting from the application of any of the information provided by this guide. This disclaimer applies to any damages or injury caused by the use and application, whether directly or indirectly, of any advice or information presented, whether for breach of contract, tort, negligence, personal injury, criminal intent, or under any other cause of action.

You agree to accept all risks of using the information presented inside this book. You need to consult a professional medical practitioner in order to ensure you are both able and healthy enough to participate in this program.

Table of Contents

Introduction 6
   Yin and Yang Philosophy 6

Chapter 1: Star Recipe 11
   Ingredients (For 10 servings) 13
   Method 13
   Secret Tips 14

Chapter 2: Red Easter Eggs 15
   Ingredients (For 10 servings) 15
   Method 15

Chapter 3: The Most Versatile Meat 17
   Ingredients (For 1 serving) 18
   Method 19
   Secret Tips 20

Chapter 4: The Wonderful Women's Herb 23
   Ingredients (For 1 serving) 24
   Method 25
   Secret Tips 25

Chapter 5: Soups To Restore Your Health 27
   Ingredients (For 1 serving) 27
   Method 28
   Secret Tips 28

Chapter 6: Nutritious Lactation Secret Recipe 37
   Ingredients (For 2 servings) 38
   Method 38
   Secret Tips 39

Chapter 7: Breakfast To Jump Start Your Day 40

- Ingredients (For 2 servings) 42
- Method 43
- Secret Tips 43

Chapter 8: Dinner's Time 45
- Ingredients (For 2 servings) 46
- Method 47
- Secret Tips 47

Chapter 9: Booster Recipes 52
- Ingredients 52
- Method 52
- Secret Tips 52

Chapter 10: Glossary 53
- Glossary of Chinese Herbs 53
- Glossary of Chinese Medical Terms 57

Conclusion 60

Check Out Other Books 62

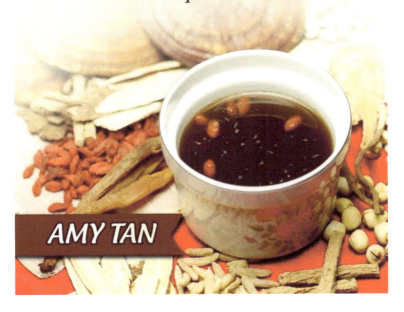

Introduction

According to Chinese tradition, after giving birth the new mother is expected to be in confinement for 30 to 40 days to recuperate from the fatigue of pregnancy. During this time, she is advised to stay at home and to avoid the outdoors. Cold, wind and dirty air, in addition to the tiredness experienced, are believed to exert a bad effect on her immediate health and later life as well. After childbirth, a woman is believed to be depleted of her Yang energy and be in a state of "blood deficiency". So she has to consume more 'hot' (Yang) foods to restore her 'cold' (Yin) bodily state. Yin and Yang affect and control each other, according to Chinese philosophy. Good health means the proportions of Yin and Yang are relatively balanced.

Yin and Yang Philosophy

Chef Martin Yan says the Yin and Yang philosophy "is one the Chinese follow not just in the preparation and cooking of food, but everyday life. For instance, if you love certain things, you learn always to watch out that you do not have too much of one thing -- even exercise, even making money, even success. If somebody is too successful, making too much money, then they have lost sight of who they are, of the family values. They don't have time to spend with the parent or with the children. So the idea of Yin and Yang is a practiced philosophy where people learn to have a better-balanced life. And food is the same.

When you go to a Chinese restaurant, when you order and prepare Chinese food, you got to watch out. You don't want to have too many deep fried dishes. You don't want too many dishes all with meat. You want to balance the meat with the vegetable dish, and you want to balance the sweet and sour with some lighter fare. You want to balance deep fried dishes with steamed dishes. It's all about balance."

Yin Foods –banana, water melon, pineapple ,bean sprouts, chicken egg white, cabbage, cucumber, duck, tofu, crab and water

Neutral Foods –apple, papaya, chicken egg yolk, duck, pork, brown rice, pumpkin, fungus, honey and dates

Yang Foods –mango, mandarin orange, grape, cherry, black currant, peaches, beef, chicken, eggs, ginger, glutinous rice, sesame oil, mushrooms, longan, vinegar and wine

Food as Medicine

For centuries, the Chinese have believed that food should be eaten not only for nutrition but also as medicinal remedy. They knew that eating the proper foods boosted the immune system, prevented health problems, helped fight diseases and increased a person's longevity. The five major organ systems of the body: the heart, liver, spleen/pancreas, lungs and kidneys required to match the nutrition needs of these five flavors: sweet, sour, bitter, pungent, and salty.

The correct ingredient proportions must be adhered to, in the preparation of each dish or soup to ensure full nutritional value. Chinese herbs are used in some of these secret recipes to speed up the healing process. Many of the plants used in these secret recipes, including ginger, Chinese herbs and fungus, have properties of preventing and alleviating various illnesses. Traditional Chinese herbal medicine has been practiced for over 5000 years. Chinese herbs are used to counter balance the symptoms of disease and to restore order.

Just like foods, Chinese herbs are also categorized as hot or cold, dry or damp. Chinese theory believes that food and herbs have a directional effect on energy flows (Qi) within our body. The other fundamental substance is 'essence'(Jing) or 'blood' (Xue).Herbs and foods are used to strengthen these vital substances to maintain health. The secret recipes in this book contain balanced meals to ensure an overall effect that is neutral.

The secret recipes in this book are contributed from the wisdom of Chinese ancient scholars and traditional Chinese midwives and each recipe has been thoroughly tested in our kitchen. The wise Chinese midwives say women after 40 have sagging breasts and skin that "looks and feels like tree bark" because they did not follow the postpartum confinement rules. These Chinese midwives add that such women have bone problems or gynecological illnesses because they did not eat properly after giving birth. Chinese midwives are also known as (aka) Confinement nannies are traditionally hired by the Chinese to help care for both the mother and baby during the convalescent month after birth. They are usually middle-aged women with great knowledge about post-natal matters by virtue of their experience.

Sitting The Month

Traditionally, the Chinese have given mothers 30 to 40 days to recover in what is called "sitting the month". New mothers spend the first 30 days after childbirth doing little more than sleeping, receiving special treats and getting used to their new role in life both physically and psychologically. There could be wisdom in this practice. Many complications can arise if the new mother does not take care of herself during this period.

Going on diet too soon to lose weight could increase the chance of having complications and weaken the body's constitution, which could result in serious health problems in later years. The tradition of "sitting the month" can be traced back to the Chin dynasty (221-206 B.C.) though it was not until the Sung dynasty (960-1279) that the term was first used. Some believe that the custom originated as a way to thank daughters-in-law for continuing the family line.

During the first month, new mothers, who often shouldered many household burdens, could not only rest but got priority at mealtimes. In addition, mothers-in-law prepared a variety of dishes, including pork kidneys and other internal organs -- regarded as expensive delicacies -- not only to build up the new mother's strength, but also to help produce sturdy descendants in the future. Strict custom dictated etiquette rules as well.

During postpartum confinement (aka "sitting the month"), women were required to remain in stuffy rooms with doors and windows completely shut, since breeze and wind were believed to cause bone problems, susceptibility to colds and headaches. Drinking plain water, bathing or washing the hair was deemed detrimental to postpartum recovery as it was "cooling". The new mothers were given rice wine in place of water, for mothers who breastfeed their babies, we recommend red dates tea **(Recipe 13)** and formulated beverages.

If new mothers who can't resist the temptation to bathe and wash their hair, should do it with caution to avoid getting chilled. Add "Da Fong Cao", a Chinese herb, (scientific name: "Blumeae Balsamiferae") to warm water to remove "wind" from the body. This herb can be purchased from any Chinese herb shop. You can also replace the Chinese herb with lemon grass which is much easily available.

The key to a good postpartum confinement, according to popular lore, is avoidance of any substances with cooling properties. Drinking plain water and eating foods with "cooling" properties are strictly forbidden. Although there is still no scientific evidence that such practices are effective, neither is there evidence on the contrary. Taking the time and effort to "sit the month" may be a small price to pay to avoid possible serious health problems, which may plague a new mother later in her life.

Chapter 1: Star Recipe

For generations, Chinese families have distributed this dish to those near and dear, 12 days after the baby's birth to announce the joyous arrival. It is again served as part of a sumptuous feast when the baby is one-month-old to family, relatives and friends. The vinegar dissolves some calcium from the bones in the pork knuckles, easing absorption into the body.

The unsweetened vinegar dilutes the thick stew, and also plays an important role in stimulating the liver and gall bladder, and improving blood circulation. The liver produces bile, which is stored and released by the gall bladder to digest oil and fat.

Recipe 1 - Pig Trotter with Black Vinegar and Ginger

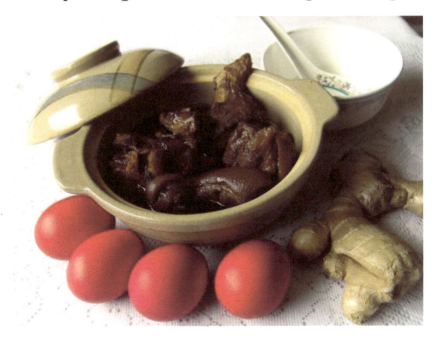

Herbs and spices present in the vinegar contain nutrients, which research shows to be anti-oxidants. Antioxidants cleanse the body of the free radicals that contribute to serious illnesses.

The Chinese have been using rice to make vinegar for over 2000 years. There are three types of Chinese rice vinegar: white, red and black.

Chinese White or Pale Amber Vinegar as its name implies, this is a pale-colored rice vinegar frequently used in sweet and sour dishes and as a dressing for raw vegetables. It should be used in moderation.

Chinese Red Vinegar is made from red rice, this sweet vinegar is used for two reasons: to cut the richness of certain foods and to highlight the sweetness in soups, stews and seafood. It is used as a dip for oysters on the half shell, steamed dumplings and fried prawns.

Chinese Black Vinegar is the type of vinegar commonly used for this star recipe. It is believed to restore strength. In Southern China it is made into a tonic and given to women after childbirth. This dark brown vinegar has a rich, sweet flavor similar to a Spanish sherry vinegar or Italian balsamic vinegar.

 Like the red vinegar it is used to balance excessively rich or sweet dishes. It can be bought either plain or in a variety of extra-sweet, seasoned versions and even with herbs added.

Recipe 1 - Pig Trotter with Black Vinegar and Ginger

To help a new mother recover her strength, traditionally she was fed the calcium and protein-rich **Pig Trotter with Black Vinegar and Ginger**. Each ingredient in this stew is a key component of its fortifying properties. Sugars, which are present in the form of glucose and fructose, replenish energy. Moreover, it tastes great!

Ingredients (For 10 servings)

Group 1

- 1 pig's trotter (1kg), cut into serving pieces

Group 2

- 1kg old ginger, skinned and smashed lightly

Group 3

- 750g black vinegar
- 1.5kg water
- 50g sesame oil

Group 4

- 300g brown sugar
- 2 teaspoons salt

Group 5

- 10 hardboiled eggs

Method

1. Heat wok with sesame oil and add ginger, fry at low heat till golden brown and aromatic.

2. Dish out and transfer ginger into a clay pot and add **Group 3** ingredients and bring to boil.

3. Add **Group 4** ingredients to taste.

4. Blanch trotter pieces in boiling water for a while. Remove and shake off excess water.

5. Add trotters into stew and boil for 2 hours until trotters are tender and soft.

6. Add hardboiled eggs before serving.

Secret Tips

1. You can prepare the stew (**Method 1 to 4**) one month before childbirth. When adding **Group 3** ingredients, add vinegar followed by water. The stew can keep up to 2 to 3 months if no sugar is added. Re-boil it twice a week to kill any bacteria in the mixture to prevent mould forming.

2. One day before distributing dish, heat the stew and carry out **Method 5 and 6**.

3. The dish will keep for 2 days before serving. The stew becomes thicker and trotters will taste even better.

Chapter 2: Red Easter Eggs

Eggs were considered a delicacy in traditional China and were usually reserved for special occasions or guests. One month after a child's birth, hardboiled eggs symbolizing fertility were dyed red for good luck and given to family, friends and relatives. Their presence was seen as having honored the child's birth.

Eggs are full of protein especially albumin and globulin, and vitamins A, B1, B2, B6, B12, D and E, minerals such as calcium, phosphorus and iron. Thus they help nurture the blood because blood serum contains large amount of protein, the two major groups being albumin and globulin, and iron.

How do you make the red eggs? Before you make the red eggs, you must learn how to prepare a perfect hardboiled egg.

Recipe 2-Perfect Hardboiled Eggs

Ingredients (For 10 servings)

- 10 eggs
- 1/2 teaspoon salt
- Water

Method

1. Place eggs in a pot.
2. Add salt in the pot
3. Cover the eggs with cold water.

4. Put the pot on the stove and bring to a boil

5. Remove from heat and wait for 20 minutes.

6. Pour off hot water and run cold water over eggs to stop cooking process.

Red Easter Eggs

Ingredients

- 10 perfect hard boiled eggs
- 2 teaspoons red dye powder
- 1 teaspoon of vinegar

Method

1. Mix the red dye with one cup of hot water in a bowl.

2. Blend evenly, add vinegar and mix well.

3. Dip one egg at a time into the red dye mixture.

4. Roll egg around to obtain an even color on the shell.

5. Leave eggs to cool & dry.

Chapter 3: The Most Versatile Meat

The chicken is the most versatile of meats .Chicken is roasted, steamed, baked, boiled, stir-fried, deep-fried, and pan-fried. It is served hot, cold, or at room temperature. No part of the chicken is wasted from its bones to its skin to its feet, which is a Chinese delicacy to its butt, which is a great source of protein, iron and calcium.

Its taste is sweet, its nature is warm, and it benefits the spleen and stomach. Chicken meat nourishes the '*Qi* ', blood, kidneys and essence. It is used to treat blood deficiency, emaciation, heart palpitations, dizziness and persistent illness.

Recipes 3 to 9 show how chicken can be prepared for a mother after childbirth -- fried, roasted or in soups.

Recipe 3 - Fried Chicken with Sesame Oil

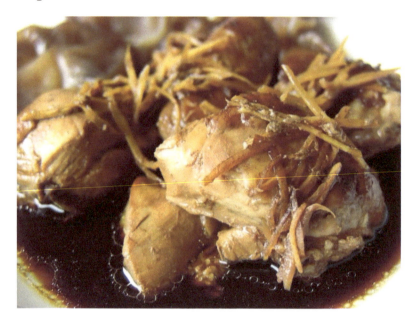

This dish benefits the large intestines, prevents a woman's breasts from sagging after childbirth, reduces swelling in the legs, stimulates hair and muscle growth, and prevents skin infection.

Ingredients (For 1 serving)

Group 1

- 300g chicken
- 1/4 teaspoon salt
- 1/2 teaspoon sugar

Group 2

- 3g mushrooms

- 30g straw mushroom
- 3g black fungus

Group 3
- 20g ginger
- 20g sesame oil

Group 4
- 6 tablespoons rice wine

Group 5
- 1 tablespoon dark soy sauce
- 1 tablespoon sugar

Method

1. Cut the chicken into pieces and add **Group 1** seasoning. Keep for 20 minutes.
2. Soak **Group 2** ingredients for 30 minutes and slice the mushroom and black fungus.
3. Shred the ginger from **Group 3** ingredients.
4. Fry **Group 3** ingredients, add **Group 1,2 and 4** ingredients and cover for 3 minutes till chicken is cooked.
5. Finally add **Group 5** ingredients and stir well.

Secret Tips

1. Black sesame oil is the top choice in this dish for medicinal purpose. White sesame oil is the second choice.

2. Raw oil is "cold" in nature, so it is advisable to ensure the sesame oil is "cooked", that is heated first.

Sesame oil

Chinese women still consume sesame oil during postpartum confinement. Sufficient intake of sesame oil during the postpartum confinement is believed to help in the contraction of the womb, which had been severely stretched during childbirth. It also helps to eliminate the remaining blood clots and stimulate lactation.

Sesame oil was rarely consumed in ancient China as it was considered a luxury. It was used as seasoning by the rich and in restaurants. Commoners could not afford sesame oil as a daily seasoning, but could only have it during the postpartum confinement.

From a scientific point of view, sesame oil has high nutritional content and energy. Every 50g of sesame oil contains about 500 kilocalories, 16g of protein, 53g of fats. It is suitable for long-term consumption by those who live in cold areas and those who are weak and poor in health. Sesame oil also contains minerals such as calcium, phosphorous, iron and magnesium, and vitamins such as B1, B2 and E. Vitamin E is an antioxidant that helps to prevent the body from aging and contracting cancer.

Sesame oil is cold-pressed from sesame seeds. It comes in two varieties: non-toasted sesame oil and toasted sesame oil. Non-toasted sesame oil has a slight nutty flavor and is especially good for frying. Toasted sesame oil has a stronger flavor and aroma and is widely used as a seasoning. Both varieties are a good source of polyunsaturated fat. The main fatty acid in sesame oil is Linoleic acid, a polyunsaturated fatty acid. The human body is unable to produce linoleic acid on its own. Hence it is one of the most important essential fatty acids to be obtained through diet.

Recipe 4 - Roasted Dang Gui Chicken with Honey

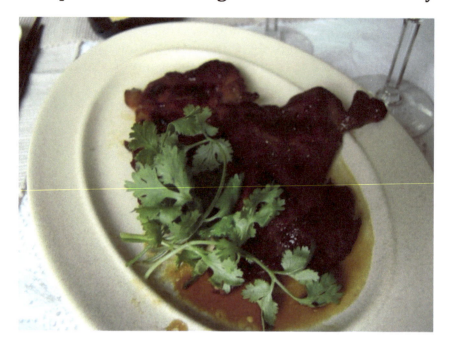

Chapter 4: The Wonderful Women's Herb

Dang Gui is a good and wonderful herb for women. Chinese mothers normally start with small doses of Dang Gui 10 to 14 days after giving birth. However, expectant mothers should avoid taking this herb, as it is believed that its consumption may increase the risk of a miscarriage. Scientifically known as Angelica Sinensis, Dang Gui is the roots of a fragrant perennial herb.

It is highly aromatic and is sold in flat, irregular pieces with brown-spotted oil cavities. It is a general herb and known as the great tonic for all female deficiencies. It activates the flow of blood and relieves painful and abnormal menstruation and premenstrual syndrome.

Dang Gui also enriches the blood and promotes circulation. Dang Gui has many other functions that are related it to its blood building and blood moving properties. It is used to treat tinnitus, arthritis, blurred vision and palpitations. Dang Gui has also been proven to enhance immunity by stimulating the production and activity of white blood cells. Moreover, it stimulates the appetite, improves muscle tone, kills bacteria, moistens the intestines and is a cure for loose bowel. Do not use this herb if you have diarrhea as Dang Gui also nourishes the intestines and treats constipation.

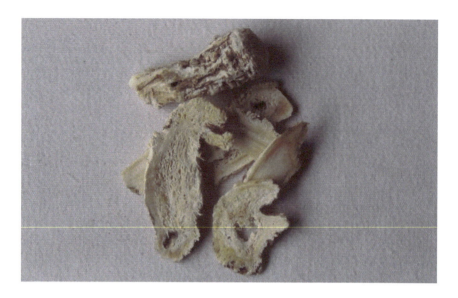

Dang Gui

Recipe 4 - Roasted Dang Gui Chicken with Honey

This dish is improvised from the Western food in the fine dining except without the Dang Gui and ginger juice. It is modified with the addition of Dang Gui powder to help activate the circulation of blood and ginger to warm the stomach. Slicing Dang Gui, heating the slices in an oven for a while, removing them and then grinding the slices into powder, makes Dang Gui powder.

Ingredients (For 1 serving)

Group 1

- 300g de-boned chicken thighs
- 1/2 teaspoon salt
- 3 teaspoons sugar

- 2 teaspoons ginger juice
- 1 teaspoon light soy sauce
- 1 teaspoon dark soy sauce
- 3 teaspoons Dang Gui (Chinese Angelica) powder

Group 2
- 3 teaspoons honey

Method

1. Mix Group 1 ingredients and let chicken season for 1 hour.
2. Place chicken on a wire rack.
3. Set oven temperature to 200°C and roast for 7 minutes, remove and apply honey and put chicken back into oven and roast for another 3 minutes.
4. Flip the chicken over and repeat step 3 to give the other side a chance to brown.
5. Serve hot.

Secret Tips

1. One secret to really flavorful, juicy roast chicken is to extend the seasoning time. You can leave the chicken in the fridge for 1 day to season.
2. Apply some oil on wire rack to prevent the chicken sticking onto the rack.

Honey

In ancient Greece, honey was used as a dressing for wounds, skin and hair care treatment. It is also a wonderful source of energy as it adds few calories. Moreover, it is an excellent source of carbohydrate for post-workout muscle recuperation and energy repletion. Honey contains polyphenols, which act as antioxidants.

Light and Dark Soy Sauce

Both light and dark sauces are used here in most of the recipes. Dark soy sauce is thicker and darker in color due to longer brewing and the addition of caramel. It is used to add a rich, dark-brown color to the appearance of this dish and it is also not quite as salty as light soy sauce. Light sauce is added to enhance taste. Soy sauce was prepared by the Chinese and introduced to Japan about a thousand years ago. Devised as a means of preserving food, the first soy sauce was in all probability liquid bean sauces. Soy sauce is a naturally fermented product made from ground soybeans, wheat, flour and yeast.

After fermentation has begun, salt water equal to the original weight of the soybeans is added. The soybeans are then being sunned for a period of one year. The resultant mash is allowed to age. When sufficiently mellow, it is strained and bottled. When choosing soy sauce, we have to be aware that they are traditionally brewed or produced synthetically from hydrolyzed vegetable protein and caramel. You can't tell by visual the difference between the real and imitation soy sauce. Therefore it is important to read the label and check the contents and how it is manufactured.

Enjoying this book so far? I'd love it for you to share your thoughts and post a quick review on Amazon!

Click here to leave a review on Amazon.com.

Chapter 5: Soups To Restore Your Health

Soup has been designed to restore the Yang forces. Chicken, a warming or Yang food, may be combined with a number of other ingredients, such as black fungus, Dang Gui, Ling Zhi and a combination of Chinese herbs.

Recipe 5 - Chicken with Ginger Juice and Wine Soup

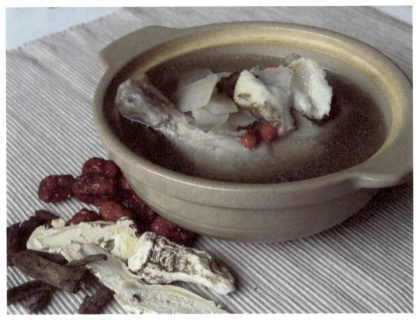

Ingredients (For 1 serving)

Group 1
- 300g black-bone chicken

Group 2
- 100g ginger juices

Group 3
- 100g wine

Group 4
- 1/4 teaspoon salt

Method
1. Remove the skin of the black-bone chicken.
2. Place all ingredients except salt into a double boiler.
3. Boil for 2 hours.
4. Add salt to taste.

Secret Tips
1. If you don't have a double boiler, this technique can be achieved by placing a metal bowl or smaller pot inside a larger pot of boiling water.
2. You need about 180g of ginger to produce 100g of juice.

Black - Bone Chicken

In all the soup recipes, the chicken can be replaced with the black-bone chicken.

Recipes 5 to 9, use a 1.5kg chicken.

Medical research shows that the black chicken or black bone chicken is rich in black pigments, which helps in anemia. The iron content in its serum and liver are two times more than a farm chicken's; its vitamin A content is ten times more than an eel's; its vitamin B2 is 1.8 times more than that found in the liver of a cow, and its iron content is ten times more than in spinach (100g of spinach contains 3mg of iron).

It has low sugar content, possesses alkaline pH and amazingly, contains DHA (docosahexaenoic acid) and EPA (Eicosapentaenoic acid). These cannot be found in other animal meat like beef, mutton or pork. It says the Taihe Old Chicken is a tonic and nourishing food to treat women's diseases and makes a precious medicinal dish when cooked with herbs.

To identify a black-bone chicken, just examine its tongue. A black tongue indicates it is a black-bone chicken. Also spelled as Black-boned Chicken, it is called Silkie Bantam in the United States. The skin of the chicken is black and hence its name. We use a double boiler to boil it for two hours. Double boiling is a simple technique used by Chinese cooks where a food is cooked slowly within a closed container. The result is a very clear, intense broth.

Recipe 6 - Chicken with Black Fungus in Wine Soup

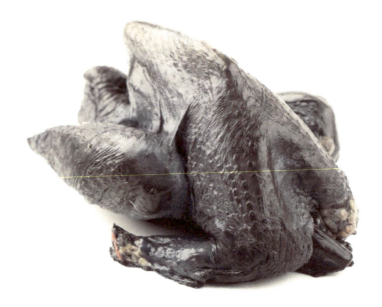

Chinese practitioners also recommend this recipe for the treatment of scanty and pro-longed postpartum discharge, dizziness, abdominal pain, and pain during urination. They recommend consumption of this dish with a meal once a day for five days as one course. If necessary, it has to be repeated with one more course for complete recovery.

Ingredients (For 1 serving)

Group 1

- 300g de-boned chicken thighs
- 1/2 teaspoon salt

Group 2
- 30g shredded ginger

Group 3
- 10g black fungus

Group 4
- 30g peanut
- 1 teaspoon salt

Group 5
- 200g chicken bones
- 500g water

Group 6
- 10g sesame oil

Group 7
- 1/2 teaspoon salt
- 30g wine

Method
1. Wash chicken, remove skin and fat.
2. Mix **Group 1** ingredients and season for 10 minutes.
3. Soak black fungus for 30 minutes until soft, rinse and cut into thin strips.
4. Apply this step if raw peanut is used. Add **Group 4**

ingredients into boiling water and soak for 30 minutes and drain dry.

5. Prepare chicken stock by adding **Group 4** ingredients into **Group 5** ingredients and boil for 30 minutes.
6. Heat wok with sesame oil, add shredded ginger, shredded black fungus, chicken and chicken stock and fry for about 5 minutes.
7. Add **Group 7** ingredients to taste.
8. Serve and eat all ingredients in the dish with soup.

Secret Tips

1. In the preparation of soups, always add salt last. The amount of salt added depends on the preference of each individual. For those who don't like the soup to be salty or cannot take much salt, you may use less salt.

Black fungus

Black fungus, also known as wood ear fungus, is sweet in taste. Its nature is neutral, and it benefits the lung, stomach, and liver. It is used for dry cough, dry throat and mouth, and for other symptoms of dryness. It is good for blood circulation, cleansing the womb, and to ease excessive menstrual bleeding. It is more therapeutic than white fungus, also known as cloud ear fungus.

Recipe 7- Chicken with Dang Gui Soup

Ingredients (For 4 servings)

Group 1

- 30g Dang Gui (Chinese Angelica)
- 20g He Shou Wu (*Polygonum Multiflorum*)
- 10g Ba Ji Tian (Morinda)
- 10g Da Zao (Jujube dates)
- 10g Gou Qi Zi (Lycii berries)

Recipe 8 - Chicken with Ling Zhi Soup

If you have flu, the most important function that Dang Gui has in this chicken soup is to disperse cold and treat pain associated with cold damp.

Ingredients (For 4 servings)

Group 1

- 5g Ling Zhi (Reishi or Ganoderma)
- 20g Dang Shen (Codonopsis)
- 10g Ren Shen Xu (Ginseng roots)
- 10g Gou Qi Zi (Lycii berries)
- 10g Da Zao (Jujube dates)

Ling Zhi

Ganoderma Lucidum--known in China as Ling Chi (Mushroom of Immortality) and in Japan as reishi--is one of the most famous medicinal mushrooms. In traditional Chinese medicine, reishi is considered to be in the highest class of tonics for promoting longevity. There are at least six varieties: red, purple, black, white, green and yellow. Red and black Ling Zhi is most common and purple is extremely rare.

The health benefits of Ling Zhi are extremely broad. It is most famous for its anti-aging property and strengthening of the immune system. Nowadays most of the Ling Zhi available is cultivated because the wild ones are extremely difficult to find.

Ling Zhi also treats hypertension and coronary heart disease, AIDS, cancer, asthma, rheumatism, insomnia, stress, high blood pressure, liver diseases, fatigue and lack of strength.

Recipe 9 - Du Zhong Bu Yao Soup

This particular soup was traditionally used to strengthen the liver and kidneys. It is not advisable for pregnant women as it uses Niu Xi, which invigorates blood circulation and clears stagnant blood. This will affect the growth of the fetus as it receives all the necessary nutrition, oxygen, and life support from the mother through the blood vessels in the umbilical cord.

Ingredients (For 4 servings)
Group 1

- 10g Niu Xi (Achyranthes)
- 10g Du Zhong (Eucommia)

- 10g Bei Qi (also known as Huang Qi, Astragalus roots)
- 15g Dang Shen (Codonopsis)
- 10g Gou Qi Zi (Lycii berries)
- 20g Long Yan Rou (Longan berries)

Method for Recipe 7 to 9

1. Remove the skin of the chicken and rinse in hot water for a minute.
2. Rinse in cold water and drain water off the chicken.
3. Place **Group 1** ingredients into ceramic crock-pot and add 3kg of water.
4. Cover the crock-pot and bring to boil.
5. When the stock is boiling, put in chicken and boil for about 3 hours.
6. Add salt to taste.

Secret Tips

1. The ingredients in Recipe 7 to 9 can be easily purchased from shops selling Chinese medicines and herbs.

Du Zhong

Du Zhong or Cortex Eucommiae Ulmoidis is the main ingredient in Chinese remedies for back pain. Bu Yao means "strengthen the waist". It is combined with other herbs such as Niu Xi for treating pain in the back and lower limbs. This bark of a superior herb was mostly cultivated and has been prized as a potent health tonic for over three thousand years. Consumed alone, it has no side effects and is one of the best remedies for high blood pressure, lumbago and cramps during pregnancy. It is also suitable for numbness and pain in lower back and knees, headache and dizziness due to liver disorder and chronic fatigue.

Chapter 6: Nutritious Lactation Secret Recipe

This dish is best for lactating mothers who want to produce more milk for breastfeeding. Fresh fishtail boiled with half ripe papaya is said to "open up" the breast of a new mother "like a tap overflowing with milk". According to Chinese records, the sap from the papaya and protein from the fish enriches the milk glands and drinking this soup occasionally during the breastfeeding period will fill up the nursing mother's natural milk reservoirs.

Recipe 10 - Fishtail with Papaya Soup

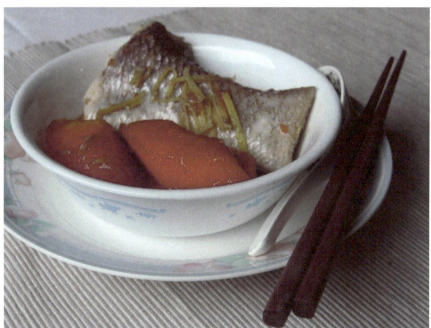

Ingredients (For 2 servings)

Group 1
- 2 papaya, (about 300g)
- 100g apple

Group 2
- 3 teaspoons oil
- 3 slices old ginger
- 1 fresh fish tail (500g)

Group 3
- 2kg boiling water

Group 4
- 3 pieces figs
- 10g almond
- 1/4 teaspoon salt

Method

1. Cut papaya and apple into cubes/wedges.
2. Heat oil & fry ginger slices, then fry fishtail for about 10 minutes.
3. Add boiling water and put all ingredients into a pot except salt and boil for about 1 hour.
4. Add salt to taste.

Secret Tips

1. While applying **Method 2** to remove fishy smell, add some liquor.

2. While applying **Method 3**, switch from high heat to medium heat. Scoop off oil on top of soup when is formed.

3. Use raw or half ripe papaya with dripping sap. This is believed to help the new mother lactate better.

4. If fishtail is not available, fish bones or fish meat may be used.

Half-Ripe Papaya

The papaya has been found to be a good source of beta-carotene. This helps prevent damage by free radicals, which might otherwise lead to some form of cancer.

Different types of enzymes, including papain , are present in papaya. Papain helps to digest the protein in food. The unripe fruit is a rich source of papain, which is vegetable pepsin and is capable of digesting protein in acid, alkaline or neutral medium. Papain also exhibits pain-relieving properties. Unripe papaya has the property of tenderizing meat. Ripe papaya, when consumed regularly, will ensure a good supply of vitamin A and C. Both ripe and unripe papaya is essential for good health.

Chapter 7: Breakfast To Jump Start Your Day

Congee is eaten throughout China as a breakfast. This simple rice soup is easily digested and assimilated. Congee requires less cooking time, from 30 minutes to one hour. It involves cooking rice with more water than usual, together with herbs and other ingredients to make rice soup.

Preferably use unpolished rice, as it is far more nutritious. It contains more B vitamins than white rice because white rice has the bran layer and the embryo of the seed removed.. It is important that the water is at a boil before rice and other ingredients are put in so that they will not sink to the bottom and burn.

Medium to medium-high heat should be maintained throughout the cooking so that the ingredients keep rising to the top and not burn. Constant stirring and keeping the lid half or fully open can prevent burning and overflowing. Hot water should be added to the cooking whenever necessary to keep the congee at the desirable thickness. The resulting congee is semi-solid, soft, easy to eat and digest.

After giving birth, a woman is often weak due to blood loss and energy used in delivering the baby. Due to blood deficiency and low energy and hence a deficiency of Yin fluids, she easily develops inflammations and other heat symptoms. The cooling, demulcent and nourishing properties of congee are therefore particularly welcome for a new mother. It is also useful for increasing a nursing mother's supply of milk.

Recipe 11- Six-Herbs Chicken Congee

The Six-Herb Chicken Congee consists of 100 g of white rice soaked in water for 2 hours. Other therapeutic properties may be added to the congee by adding the appropriate herbs and meats (in this case, chicken).

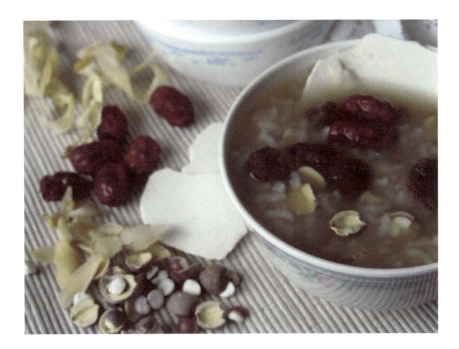

Metric weights are given throughout this book to conform to Western standards. However, Chinese herbal dosage is customarily given according to their own standard or weights and measures as follow:

- 1 fen = 0.3g approx.
- 10 fen = 1 qin = 3g approx.
- 10 qin = 1 liang = 30g approx.
- 16 liang = 1 jin = 480g approx.

Recipe 11- Six-Herbs Chicken Congee

Ingredients (For 2 servings)

Group 1
- 1/2 chicken, (about 500g)

Group 2
- 100g white rice

Group 3
- 20g Huai Shan (Chinese wild yam or Dioscorea)
- 10g Fu Shen (Poria)
- 10g Qian Shi (Euryale)
- 20g Lian Zi (Lotus seed or Nelumbo)
- 10g Bai He (Lily bulb or Lilium)
- 5g Long Yan Rou (Longan berries)
- 10g Hong Zao (Jujube dates)

Group 4
- 2kg water

Group 5
- 2 teaspoons salt

Method

1. Remove the skin of the chicken and rinse in boiling water for a minute.
2. Rinse with cold water and drain.
3. Soak white rice in water for 2 hours.
4. Wash and soak herbs in **Group 3** in water for 5 minutes.
5. Remove herbs. Put herbs and rice into water and bring to boil.
6. Add the chicken and boil for 2 hour
7. Add salt to taste

Secret Tips

1. Lower heat and simmer, uncovered for approximately 1hour or until the rice is thoroughly broken up.
2. Stir occasionally to prevent the soup from sticking and add boiling water if necessary.
3. Preferably use unpolished rice. Unpolished rice is brownish in color, less attractive looking than white rice, but the flavor is fine and it is more nutritious.

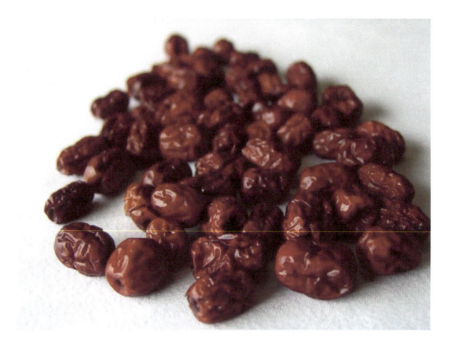

Red dates are the additional herbs added, as red dates are known to strengthen the functions of heart and lung, as well as nourish the stomach and spleen. Red dates also support normal blood pressure. They are rich in Vitamin C, which is essential for general health.

Chapter 8: Dinner's Time

Chinese myth tells of rice being a gift of animals rather than of gods. China had been visited by an especially severe period of floods. When the land had been finally drained, people came down from the hills where they had taken refuge, only to discover that all the plants had been destroyed and there was little to eat. They survived through hunting, but it was very difficult, because animals were scarce. One day the people saw a dog coming across a field, and hanging on the dog's tail were bunches of long, yellow seeds. The people planted these seeds. Rice grew, and the hunger disappeared.

Recipe 12 - Fried Rice with Egg and Ginger

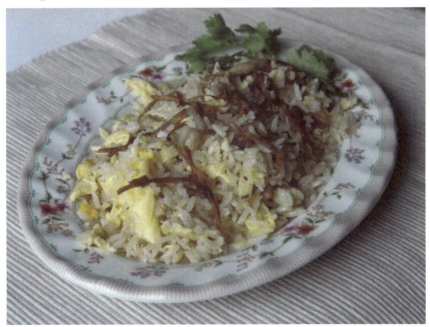

Ingredients (For 2 servings)

Group 1

- 250g white rice
- 2 slices of Dang Gui
- 10g ginger juice
- 370g water

Group 2

1. 100g chicken fillet
2. 1/2 teaspoon salt
3. 1 teaspoon sugar·
4. 1 teaspoon corn flour
5. 1/4 teaspoon pepper
6. 1/2 teaspoon sesame oil

Group 3

- 2 eggs

Group 4

- 50g Gailan

(Chinese Broccoli)

- 30g shredded ginger

Group 5

- 1/2 teaspoon salt

- 1/4 teaspoon pepper

Group 6

- Sesame oil

Method

1. Add **Group 1** ingredients into rice cooker to cook the rice.

2. Dice the chicken fillet and add the seasoning in **Group 2** ingredients.

3. Dice the Gailan from **Group 4** ingredients.

4. Fry the eggs in **Group 3** to make omelet and remove.

5. Add sesame oil and fry ginger from **Group 4** ingredients till golden yellow and scoop up the ginger.

6. Fry the seasoned chicken fillet and remove.

7. Heat the wok with 2 drops of sesame oil. Add diced Gailan and stir in the rice, omelet and chicken, and continue stirring till piping hot.

8. Season with **Group 5** ingredients and serve.

Secret Tips

1. To prepare fragrant fried rice of "restaurant quality", do this. Use a wok over high heat and stir constantly. Preferably use day-old rice because it will be drier

than fresh rice and not stick to each other. Reduce the amount of water in **Group 1** if you find the rice is wet after your first attempt.

2. 2.. In Europe and the USA, liquid eggs are commonly used. Liquid eggs are whole eggs pasteurized and frozen in bags. They are sold to hotels, airlines and bakeries for food preparation. In Singapore, there is one such factory.

Recipe 12 - Fried Sweet Shredded Pork with Spinach

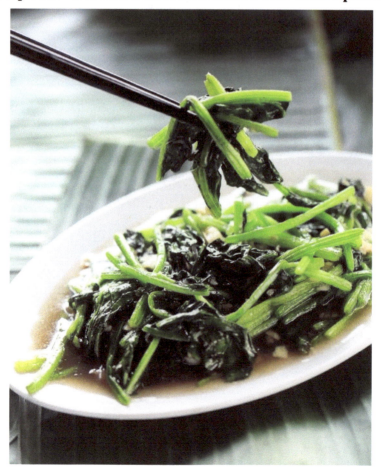

Ingredients (For 2 servings)

Group 1

- 100g shredded pork
- Pinch of salt
- •1/2 teaspoon sugar
- 1 teaspoon corn flour
- Pinch of pepper
- 1/2 teaspoon sesame oil
- 1 teaspoon oil

Group 2

- 5g mushroom

Group 3

- 5g ginseng
- 100g water

Group 4

- 300g spinach

Group 5

- 1/2 teaspoon sugar
- 1/2 teaspoon salt

- 1/2 teaspoon sesame oil

Group 6
- 1 teaspoon corn flour
- 2 teaspoons water

Group 7
- 1 teaspoon oil
- 2 slices of ginger

Method

1. Mix Group 1 ingredients and season the shredded pork for 20 minutes.
2. Soak mushroom in **Group 2** for 10 minutes and shred.
3. Boil ginseng with water from **Group 3** for 5 minutes and shred.
4. Slice off root end and half the stem of the spinach in **Group 4**.
5. Wash the spinach completely and drain leaves.
6. Heat wok, add **Group 7** ingredients. Add the seasoned pork and mushroom and cook for awhile.
7. Add **Group 5** and spinach and fry well.
8. Dish everything out of the wok and put in **Group 6** to form starch.
9. Recombine all ingredients and stir to coat spinach and serve hot.

Secret Tips

1. Korean ginseng acts faster than Chinese ginseng and is therefore more intense in nourishing Yin and Yang energies and increasing 'Qi' energy. (Please refer to glossary for Chinese medical terms).

2. For the best quality spinach, select leaves that are green and crisp, with a nice fresh fragrance. Avoid leaves that are limp, damaged, or spotted.

3. Add 5g of ginseng as its antioxidants reduce free radical in our body thereby slowing down aging.

Chapter 9: Booster Recipes

Recipe 13– Fragrant Red Dates Tea

Ingredients

- 8 red dates
- 50g black beans, pan-fried without oil
- 20g Dang Shen (Codonopsis)
- 4 slices old ginger

Method

1. Rinse all the ingredients. Put them in a pot and fill 3/4 full with hot water.
2. Boil for 2 hours.

Secret Tips

1. You can put all the ingredients into a slow cooker the night before, filling it with normal tap water. By morning, there will already be a pot of fragrant Red Dates Tea ready for consumption.
2. A simpler recipe is to add 8 red dates and 10g Long Yan Rou (Longan berries) to a pot with 3/4 full of water. Boil it for 2 hours and you can have the whole family to enjoy this pot of tea.

Chapter 10: Glossary

Glossary of Chinese Herbs

Bai He (Lillium)

Also known as Lily bulb, it is used to treat the lungs and relieve cough.

Ba Ji Tian (Morinda root)

It is used for nourishing the kidneys. Traditionally, this herb has been used for treating impotence, male or female infertility, diabetes ,premature ejaculation, and strengthening the sinews and bones. The fruit of this plant is known as Noni.

Bei Qi (Astragalus roots)

It is used to improve the action of the immune system. It is safe for many applications.

Dang Gui (Chinese Angelica)

It is used as a supplement for menstrual good health. What is not generally known is that this herb is a versatile blood tonic with many other uses.

Dang Shen (Codonopsis)

It is used as a substitute for Ginseng, in cases where the strength of Ginseng is not required. It is also a lot less expensive than Ginseng.

Da Zao (Jujube dates)

It is often added to any herbal formula that is intended to act on the digestion because it has a pleasant taste and is said to harmonize the formula. It also nourishes the blood and calms the mind - a wonderful remedy after childbirth.

Du Zhong (Eucommia)

It is the bark of the deciduous tree of the family Eucommiaceae. This nourishes the liver and kidneys, strengthens the muscles and bones and is used to stabilizing the pregnancy.

Fu Shen (Poria)

It is used to strengthen the spleen and gets rid of Dampness (Please refer to Glossary of Chinese Medical Terms) and helps digestion. It is also used to treat diarrhea, bloating and loss of appetite.

Gou Qi Zi (Lycii berries)

Also known as wolfberry, it is reputed for its ability to improve vision.

He Shou Wu (Polygonum Multiflorum)

This is used for lowering blood cholesterol, protecting against hardening of arteries, and Improve the luster and quality of hair.

Huan Shan (Dioscorea)

This is consumed to nourish the spleen and stomach. It benefits both the Yin and Yang

Of the lungs and kidneys, brightens the intellect, stimulates muscle and tendon flexibility and growth. Huan Shan is very safe and may be cooked often with food.

Jiang (Ginger)

It is widely used in these secret food recipes as it rescues the devastated Yang and expels

the interior cold (Yin). Ginger is usually regarded as safe in small amounts (up to 4 grams per day), especially as a condiment or flavoring and caution should be exercised in taking large amounts (more than 4 grams per day).Ask for professional advice before Ginger preparations during pregnancy.

Lian Zi (Nelumbo)

Also known as Lotus seed, this herb benefits the kidney, spleen and heart. It helps to regulate blood pressure and relieve numbness and aching near the waist and knees. It is also used to treat weak sexual function in men and leucorrhoea in women. The seed also has calming properties that alleviates restlessness, insomnia and palpitations.

Ling Zhi (Ganoderma)

It is used as a stimulant for the immune system and is known for its anti-aging properties.

Long Yan Rou (Longan berries)

Directly translated, it means "Dragon Eye Flesh". It is a sweet and succulent fruit, which benefits the heart and spleen. It is used for nourishing blood and calming the mind. A simplified version of red dates tea is to add 20g of longan berries with 8 red dates, fill with ¾ full pot of hot water and boil for 20 minutes.

Niu Xi (Achyranthes)

It is used to vitalize blood in the lower body. It is therefore used in formulas for leg pain, foot pain and low back pain. Do not use Niu Xi during pregnancy.

Qian Shi (Euryale)

Also known as fox nut, it is used to strengthen the kidney and spleen. It helps to regulate blood pressure and relieve numbness and aching near the waist and knees.

Glossary of Chinese Medical Terms

Dampness

This refers to abnormal body fluids, which become thick and cause disharmony and disease.

Jing (Essence)

Essence (a Yin characteristic) is that aspect of the body that is the basis for all growth, development and sexuality. Congenital Essence is that part of the body's Essence that is inherited from the parents.

After birth this Essence, which is akin to an inborn constitution, determines each of our growth patterns.

Congenital Essence can never be replaced if lost, but can be supplemented by acquired Essence, which is derived from food. Essence also has the narrow meaning of semen.

Qi (Energy)

It signifies a tendency, a movement, something on the order of energy. There are two main aspects of Qi. On the one hand, Qi is thought of as matter without form. When this substance is diseased, certain symptoms appear such as a chill or rheumatic aches and pains. Qi is also a term for the functional, active aspect of the body.

Xue (Blood)

Although the red liquid that circulates throughout the body is called blood in Western medicine, it is only part of the Chinese conception of Blood. In addition to being a substance, Blood is also regarded as a force, a level of activity in the body which is involved with the sensitivity of the sense organs, as well as at a deep level of the body in the progression of febrile diseases. The major function of Blood is to carry nourishment to all parts of the body.

Yin and Yang

Yin and Yang represent the two opposing forces or the two opposite ends of life and its manifestation and experience. For example, night and day, summer and winter, wet and dry, hot and cold, etc.

Yin is night and Yang is day. Night is resting and restoring; day is moving and growing. Night and day control the life of living organisms on earth. Without either one, life does not exist. But when either one becomes too dominating, it causes imbalance.

In Chinese medicine, health is represented as a balance of Yin and Yang. Good health means the proportions of Yin and Yang are relatively balanced.

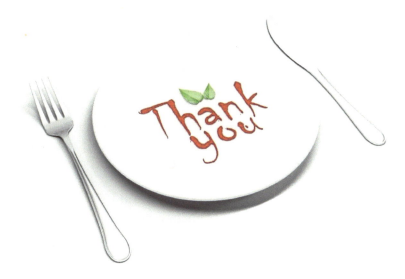

If you enjoyed this book or received value from it in any way, then I'd like to ask you for a favor: would you be kind enough to leave a review for this book on Amazon? It'd be greatly appreciated!

Click here to leave a review on Amazon.com.

Conclusion

In this instructive new mother's guide, we condense thousands of years of accumulated wisdom into readable and accessible form, highlighting one very important aspect of this invaluable tradition. The extreme impact of childbearing on the human body, with its possible negative, long-term effects on a woman's health, has customarily been treated with lengthy postpartum confinement (aka "sitting the month"), and a special postpartum diet.

In Chinese culture, "an ounce of prevention is worth a pound of cure" is not just a saying preached to the accident-prone, but the key principle of mainstream medical practice. Preventative medicine plays an essential role in every person's health regimen. Ancient wisdom passed down from generation to generation emphasizes the interrelated nature of all aspects of life and the need for balance to maintain health. Achieving this delicate balance is a serious consideration in Chinese communities, informing everyday food and lifestyle choices.

This special diet devised by wise Chinese ancestors, although they did not have the benefit of modern investigative methods or knowledge of specific chemical interactions or vitamins, zeroed-in on the very nutrient-dense foods needed to meet this specific health crisis.

How would they have known that vinegar dissolves much-needed calcium from soup bones?

What special insight led them to recommend specific herbs and spices now identified as anti-oxidants that cleanse the body of free radicals?

Today, scientific and medical findings confirm the many beneficial effects of some of these food choices. Yet this knowledge was somehow intuitively grasped and incorporated into a comprehensive health system centuries ago.

These secret recipes are classic and updated, all home-tested, in sync with the core principals of this venerated system.

This is a book for all recovering new mothers and the people who care for them.

Check Out Other Books

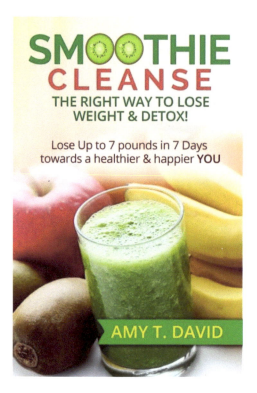

ASN:B00YJO2U88

http://www.amazon.com/SMOOTHIE-CLEANSE-RIGHT-WEIGHT-DETOX-ebook/dp/B00YJO2U88